MW00785122

Am I
Crazy?

LESLEY ANN FEIN MD, MPH

Copyright © 2022 Lesley Ann Fein MD, MPH
All rights reserved
First Edition

Fulton Books
Meadville, PA

Published by Fulton Books 2022

ISBN 978-1-63860-506-5 (paperback)
ISBN 978-1-63860-507-2 (digital)

Printed in the United States of America

I am a rheumatologist, fascinated by the relationship between infections that trigger other diseases similar to rheumatoid arthritis, lupus, multiple sclerosis, Parkinson's disease, Alzheimer's disease, fibromyalgia, psychiatric diseases, and Amyotrophic Lateral Sclerosis, to name only a few. I often see people at the end of their rope after many doctors have told them there is nothing wrong or have failed treatment for these other diseases, and after doing research, they believe that they have an underlying infection. By the time they see me, they invariably have concluded that they must be crazy! That is why I thought this title was apt for this publication.

Living on the East Coast, where tick-borne infections are an epidemic, it is common to find one of these infections after reviewing a new patient's medical records, asking many questions, reviewing testing I order, and performing a thorough physical examination.

I am stating that tick-borne infections are an epidemic because every person one meets knows someone who has been diagnosed with Lyme disease, and none of my patients with CDC positive test have been reported to the CDC. There is the law requiring a laboratory that finds a CDC positive test to notify the local health department. The health department then sends a form to both the patient and their doctor to fill out pertinent information. After that, the case is sent to the CDC for reporting as a definite case of Lyme disease.

In New Jersey, over the past thirty years I have been in private practice, I have very rarely been contacted by the health department. Therefore, a tiny fraction of these cases are being reported. When I sat down with members of the NJ Department of Health in a meeting facilitated by a well-known NJ senator, they were totally apathetic

3

and refused to follow very simple requests I asked: informing the public that they can purchase tick removal kits; informing the public that permethrin-treated clothing is available, inexpensive, safe, and repels ticks, greatly reducing the chance of getting bitten; informing people that they should save a tick after removal to be tested; etc. They refused! I was horrified! Their response was to tell me that I can do these things if I want to! I was outraged!

I have been very involved in following the research regarding Lyme and other tick-borne infections, the overlap with fibromyalgia and ME/CFS. And I became a rheumatologist because my interest was piqued when the original doctors from Yale Univeristy came to Mount Sinai Hospital in NYC, where I was a medical resident, and presented the first cases of Lyme triggering autoimmune diseases such as RA, MS, etc. This was fascinating to me, and I decided to make it my life's work. I attended the first Lyme conference at Yale in about 1984 and became an avid follower of the research ever since.

I am writing this book for two reasons. The first is to update both clinicians and patients on the recent research in this field. The reason it is important to have something accessible to clinicians is that even it is now thirty years after Lyme disease was discovered, both medical schools and internship/residency programs continue to misrepresent the complexity of tick-borne infections. The result is doctors who have not been taught anything about the true research in this field are failing their patients by not recognizing and treating them correctly.

The second reason is to educate the public so that you under-stand the basics, as well as the research in this field, so that you can be advocates for your own diagnosis and treatment.

Research regarding this topic is evolving at a rapid rate, making it difficult to keep updated.

I am covering each disease separately and then getting into how they trigger autoimmune diseases, fibromyalgia, and/or myalgic encephalomyelitis (previously called chronic fatigue syndrome), as well as informing you that chronic pain and inflammation *can* result in depression and more serious psychiatric illnesses.

Lyme Disease

*B*orrelia burgdorferi, the first bacterium identified by Willy Burgdorfer, was the first bacterium known to trigger multiple autoimmune diseases at that time, including rheumatoid arthritis, systemic lupus erythematosus, and multiple sclerosis.

This fascinated me from an intellectual perspective because it is counterintuitive to allow your own immune system to attack itself. Since then, other multiple autoimmune diseases have been associated with both bacteria and viruses.

Over the past thirty-plus years, the research about the sophistication of the bacterium itself plus the multitude of new species of *Borrelia* has flourished, yet most of the medical community have not taught this in medical school or medical residencies and receive no education to enable them to deal with the complex clinical presentations of the myriad of tick-borne infections.

Doctors who are interested in learning need to educate themselves, and unfortunately, sick patients are required to navigate their way through the politically charged and contradictory information available on the internet.

This is intended to simplify the facts without discussion about the controversy. This is an infection that is associated with more controversy than any other. The reason for this is that it can manifest in so many different ways that patients get lost running from one specialist to another with no diagnosis.

It is true that it begins as an infection. However, many people are not aware that they have been bitten by a tick in the first place. When they get symptoms ranging from joint pains, neurological symptoms, headaches, to psychiatric symptoms, they see all the various specialists, and no one thinks of Lyme disease. Thirty percent of people infected with Lyme get hearing or inner ear symptoms, so they end up at an ENT specialist. Forty percent get palpitations and end up seeing cardiologists, etc. Brain inflammation associated with Lyme disease can cause serious depression, anxiety, "Lyme rage," and overt psychosis. It can also trigger OCD and ADHD.

Facts and Myths

Deer are responsible for people getting tick bites: myth.

The term *deer tick* immediately triggers an emotional response because people think that the deer in their backyard are responsible for them getting sick. This is completely false.

The main mammal reservoir is the white-footed mouse. They are able to get close enough to humans by entering their homes and transporting ticks with them. In addition, people with dogs and cats are at higher risk because their domesticated animals can transport these tiny ticks into their homes on their fur.

Domesticated animals cannot bring ticks into the house: myth.

Another misconception is that if your dog is treated for fleas and ticks, he/she cannot transport them on their fur. This is false. Ticks grasp onto the tips of hair and will only die if they crawl all the way up to the skin of the animal. If they are carried along, attached to the hair, they will be brought inside. Ticks are extremely hardy and will remain alive with no nourishment for ten or more days. I have watched them crawling around in a container for ten days! This gives them more than enough time to find a host in the house (i.e., people)!

Most people get a rash: myth.

Most people are aware of the fact that these ticks can be as small as a pinhead when they are nymphs. They do not know that they

LESLEY ANN FEIN MD, MPH

inject anesthetic into the skin when they bite, so the person is completely unaware of being bitten. The common places they gravitate to are scalps, armpits, and groins. These are areas that would be easily missed. After they have sucked the blood of the host, they drop off and have three potential hosts before they die.

Everyone gets symptoms after a tick bite: myth.

After you are bitten, you may have absolutely no symptoms. This is seen in both humans and animals in controlled situations.

The tick must be attached for three days
before transmitting Lyme: myth.

A very common misconception is the duration of tick attachment determines whether you will be infected.

Those data came from studies on *hairless rats* in controlled laboratories, and the ticks were removed by the mouthparts. This has no relevance to human infection. Firstly, our skin is softer than rats. Secondly, we almost *never* remove ticks by the mouthparts with tweezers designed for tick removal.

I have treated Lyme patients since 1988, and I would estimate that less than 1 percent of my patients removed a tick correctly, if they were lucky enough to even see it in the first place. Most people find a tick inadvertently, often while in the shower, and grab it with their fingers to pull it off. This injects the gut contents into your bloodstream. Things like burning it with matches, rubbing alcohol, etc. are also not effective.

Please always have a tick removal kit when you go outdoors. Choose one with tweezers, photos of the different types of ticks, a small ziplock bag, and a small magnifier. If you get bitten, grab the mouthparts as close to your skin as possible, and pull the tick out. Avoid the body of the tick. Then put it in the ziplock bag, and mail it out for testing. I like this one.

8

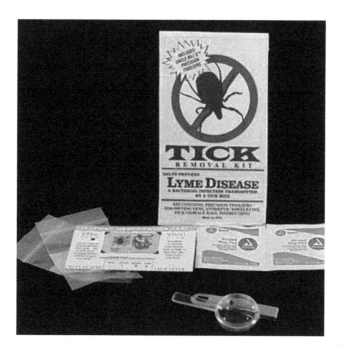

Most people get a bull's-eye rash: myth.

A rash is often not seen. Of rashes that do develop, biopsy studies done in the late 1980s, presented at the first conference at Yale and then again in the early 2000s at NYU (Dr. Andy Franks), demonstrated that *less* than 50 percent of biopsy-positive rashes are "bull's-eyes." The more common rashes range from red spots, diffuse non itchy rashes, spider bite-type rashes, hives, to pustular rashes. Some of the rashes we see are probably related to *Bartonella*, infected by the tick together with Lyme.

Early Symptoms

If people do have symptoms, they can be so vague that most people do not even seek medical care, but if they do, they are almost always told they have a viral infection. The fact is that the symptoms do usually resolve. This is also seen in animals. They become completely asymptomatic and then, three months later, get arthritis, neurological symptoms, etc. In humans, the time between infection and symptoms can be years. It can remain dormant and then become evident when the person is immunocompromised as a result of something as benign as surgery, pregnancy, or another illness or infection.

Many books are written about the clinical manifestations of Lyme disease, and I am not covering this extensively here. I have coauthored a book on this, and both Dr. Horowiz and Dr. Leigner have written extensively on the subject. As alluded to above, virtually every organ system can be involved (apart from lungs and kidneys). Suffice it to say that it can affect the brain and other parts of the nervous system, can cause arthritis called Lyme arthritis, causes a severe sleep disorder, lowers the body temperature, and can affect many hormonal pathways.

Lyme is cured after three weeks of doxycycline. Myth or truth?

Some studies suggested that early treatment is curative in 80–90 percent. This may be true. I have always given six weeks because it is a very slow-growing organism. Unfortunately, my patient population do not get treated early, and if they are, they typically receive two to three weeks of antibiotics. There are no definitive studies with adequate follow-up to support such a short course of treatment. In fact, there is a paucity of studies either way. One extremely flawed study concluded that *two* doses of doxycycline is curative.

This topic is the crux of the huge divide between the infectious diseases community, spearheaded by the IDSA, and opposing groups, the largest of which is ILADS.

Truthfully, there has been grossly insufficient funding for studies. The few prospective studies have been analyzed by Fallon et al. in "A Reappraisal of the US Clinical Trials of Post-Treatment Lyme Disease Syndrome." He concludes:

> The conclusions of this analysis of the chronic Lyme trials emphasize the benefits of repeated antibiotic therapy for patients with specific chronic symptoms. This is done as a counterbalance to the majority of published guidelines, which overlook and/or dismiss the evidence that demonstrates that additional antibiotic therapy can lead to sustained benefit. We hope that our review will lead to more carefully detailed and balanced summaries in future guidelines. However, we also wish to emphasize that while some patients do improve with repeated antibiotic therapy, other patients with persistent symptoms do not. Further, as the clinical trials also demonstrate, antibiotic therapy particularly when given intravenously can put the patient at serious risk.
>
> Biomarkers are needed that can help clinicians to discriminate in advance which patients are more likely to benefit from repeated antibiotic therapy vs. those for whom such treatment is unlikely to be beneficial. Future studies must also begin to address nonantibiotic strategies to help improve persistent symptoms. Recent serologic and CSF studies of patients with post-

treatment Lyme disease syndrome suggest that a persistently activated immune response may play a role in the pathophysiology of chronic symptoms. Clarification of whether these findings are of pathogenic relevance and whether this immune activation is due to persistent antigenic stimulation (as might occur from persistent *Borrelia*) or from a postinfectious autoimmune process would be quite beneficial to clinicians seeking to identify more effective and appropriately targeted treatments for these patients.

Since this was published, there has been a wealth of new findings that significantly affect those conclusions and must force us to reconsider how we approach treatment of Lyme disease. Dr. John Aucott recently reported that patients with "post-Lyme syndrome" have markers of persistent Lyme disease.

The bacterium causing Lyme disease has three different forms: motile form (the natural form), which most people are familiar; round bodies; and persister forms.

Round Bodies

Multiple studies have proven that the motile form of Lyme responds to antibiotics in culture by altering its form from the motile form to the "round body" form (also called cystic, cell wall-deficient, or *L* forms). This was discovered in Sweden in the 1990s but was not found in the US until Dr. Sapi et al. first cultured the bacteria and examined them. Dr. Alan MacDonald refers to these structures in his research as well. His website is www.alzheimerborreliosis.net.

When antibiotics are stopped, these forms then transform back into the motile forms, thus establishing a revolving door syndrome. This explains the frustrating conclusions from all prior prospective studies because none of them have taken this into account. The fact that patients relapsed after a course of IV Rocephin (Fallon et al.) is now explained by Sapi and her brilliant team. During IV therapy, the natural form of *B. burgdorferi* (motile form) changed into the "round bodies." If these are not treated, they are equipped with adequate DNA to change back into the motile form, thus explaining the high "relapse" rate found in these studies. *No* subsequent prospective study has been published since she presented her data, thus invalidating the prior results. She has established that the only effective treatment for these forms is Tindamax. In Europe, both Tindamax and Flagyl are effective (Brorson et al.).

Biofilms

Biofilms are a crusty shell (resembling a conch) with openings for nutrients and waste excretion, under which bacteria thrive. Dr. Sapi also elegantly presented how spirochetes create biofilms, as do many other bacterial species, making them inaccessible to antibiotics at the doses we use. She has gone further and demonstrated these biofilms in human tissues. We now know that many different bacteria can live in the same biofilm. Think of it as a well-fortified house that is heavily guarded and impossible to penetrate.

Biofilm "busters"

A lot of chatter in Lyme groups discuss the possibility of breaking up biofilms. Please do *not* think that this is a feasible option. All of our "good gut bacteria" live under biofilms, and if there was something that survived the low pH of the stomach and could potentially break open biofilms, it would decimate the gut and grossly interfere with immune function. I am hoping the audience reading this is aware that the gut is responsible for 60–80 percent of immune function. In addition, it seems implausible to the extreme that such an agent could then travel through the blood into tissues and break up biofilms in tissues!

The only two circumstances in which breaking up biofilms is safe is in the nose as treatment for antibiotic resistant *Staphylococcus* and in the lung for treatment of *Pseudomonas*.

Persister Forms / Stationary Phase

We now know from research at Northeastern University (Kim Lewis) and John Hopkins (Yin Zhang et al.) that in culture, spirochetes can stop growing after exposure to antibiotics. This is also not unique to this organism. The unique finding is that the spirochetes do not develop antibiotic resistance. If they remove the antibiotic from the culture, the organisms start to grow again and will respond to the same antibiotics used prior to them going into the stationary phase. This is the basis for their suggestion that physicians try "pulse therapy," something that has been frowned upon by the IDSA and thus the insurance companies. In the past, we had to ensure that we would *not* treat patients with this method of therapy because of the potential to create resistance in other organisms. This no longer applies in the treatment of Lyme disease.

The complicating issue is that there are many patients who are also infected with other bacterial species that do develop resistance to antibiotics, so physicians need to be cautious in this regard.

There is exciting data about combinations that are effective *in vitro* against these forms, but we yet have to prove that these are effective *in vivo*. The first triple therapy published by the Zhang group is costly and not without side effects. I have used it successfully in only one patient so far.

New studies are replete with all kinds of antibiotic combinations for these forms, but in my opinion, we need to be cautious about implementing them in humans. Anyone who wants to explore this further will find the articles referenced at the end.

Autoimmune Manifestations

If untreated, Lyme can induce many autoimmune markers in blood testing, leading to misdiagnoses. We know that people who carry the DR2 gene can develop rheumatoid arthritis, which will not respond to antibiotics even if triggered by Lyme disease.

In a retrospective study of 160 randomly selected patients in my practice, 50 percent had autoimmune markers. Most of the markers completely resolved or greatly decreased after treatment with antibiotics.

I brought up the use of Plaquenil in addition to antibiotics at conferences hosted by the Lyme Disease Foundation in the 1990s. Dr. Sam Donta took it a step further and found that Plaquenil increases the antibiotic activity of Biaxin (clarithromycin) inside cells. This combination is now used for people with Lyme disease who do not have autoimmune markers. I tend to restrict its use to only those patients with autoimmune markers or autoimmune clinical presentation. I try to limit the number of pharmaceuticals I use, if possible, especially in an era where generic medications are inadequately regulated.

Lyme triggers autoimmune manifestations in three ways:

1. It is a mitogen. That means it has the ability to stimulate the production of multiple nonspecific antibodies, some of which attack "self." In certain strains of mice, infection with *B. burgdorferi* triggers SLE, and the mice test negative for Lyme and positive for lupus. People can have the identical presentation.

16

2. Molecular mimicry. It can present your own tissue to your immune system, forcing it to make antibodies directed against your own tissue. This is not unique to Lyme.
3. Triggering autoimmune disease in genetically predisposed individuals.

The treatment of patients with both Lyme and autoimmune clinical presentations is very complex and must be decided on a case-by-case basis. Many will resolve with only antibiotics. Some will go on to have only the autoimmune presentation and will have to be treated with immunomodulators or a myriad of novel methods of treating these diseases. Some need both antibiotics plus addition of agents for immunosuppression or modulation. This would be a situation for Plaquenil to be considered as it is *not* an immunosuppressant.

Can Lyme trigger myalgic encephalomyelitis (previously known as CFS)?

Yes. Firstly, many patients with chronic Lyme disease have manifestations identical to those defined by ME. In addition, there has been a thesis whose author found Lyme disease antibodies in 50 percent of people diagnosed with ME.

Addition of the modalities of treatment used in ME must be implemented in this group to upregulate cell function, the hallmark of ME. This is *not* an easy task! These treatments are all nutraceuticals studied to enhance cell function. Many integrative/functional medicine specialists are looking for gene mutations that need to be addressed. In these cases, the underlying infections associated with ME must be sought out and addressed if the patient is to improve.

Can Lyme disease trigger fibromyalgia?

Once again, the answer is yes. Fibromyalgia (FM) is a dysfunction of neurotransmitters, which is seen in any condition causing chronic pain syndrome. The inhibitory interneurons in the spinal cord function to protect the brain from impulses generated within the pain center producing substance P. When the impulses cannot be stopped, such as is seen in any chronic pain situation, these inhibitory interneurons are unable to continue to protect the brain (referred to as the brain's *firewall*), then you are left with the "unprotected brain syndrome." This results in sensitivity to light, sound, and touch; being overwhelmed easily; anxiety; depression; and cognitive dysfunction.

Patients with FM have very abnormal responses to pain on functional MRI when compared to "normal" brains. Many of the symptoms of FM are identical to those seen in neurological Lyme disease, so it is imperative to identify and address this component as well.

The treatment is aimed at improving sleep, reducing pain, and often adding medication to restore both serotonin and norepinephrine. Addition of medications to improve concentration may be appropriate and helpful.

Specific treatment of Lyme disease cannot be discussed here. As research progresses, there are so many combinations or single agents (e.g., stevia, disulfiram) that could potentially be used. Also, each physician must decide whether to include treatments for persistent forms. In my opinion, every regimen *must* include Tindamax, which is the only prescription medication known to kill the cell wall-deficient forms or "round bodies" per Dr. Eva Sapi. The manner in which it is used is up to the treating physician, but I suggest a pulse regimen because of potential side effects. It is true that Banderol is also effective against these forms, so if a patient does not like Tindamax or develops an allergy, there is no doubt that Banderol works as well. In addition, Samento (Cat's Claw) kills the motile form of Lyme. This was published by Dr. Eva Sapi. My issue is that the correct dose is not well established for most nutraceuticals unless they have been specifically studied in humans.

I have found over the years that adding Tindamax to the regimen clearly induces a clinical response that validates the research of Dr. Eva Sapi. I typically add it one week a month. The pictures below demonstrate beautifully the typical response. In this case, the patient had been diagnosed with rheumatoid arthritis. She did not believe the diagnosis and refused immunosuppressive treatment. Her pictures clearly demonstrate how her symptoms are affected by Tindamax. The patient who filled in her joints on and off Tindamax demonstrates how important it is.

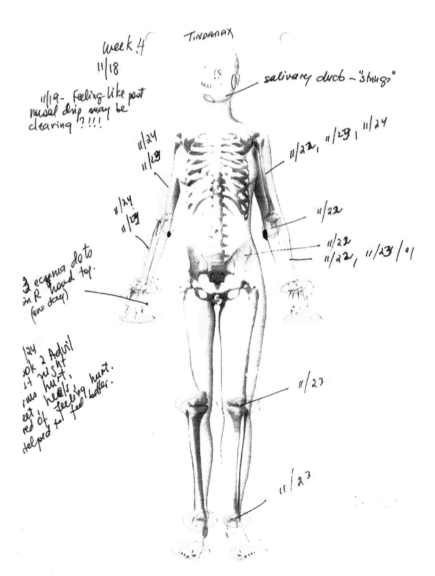

While on Tindamax

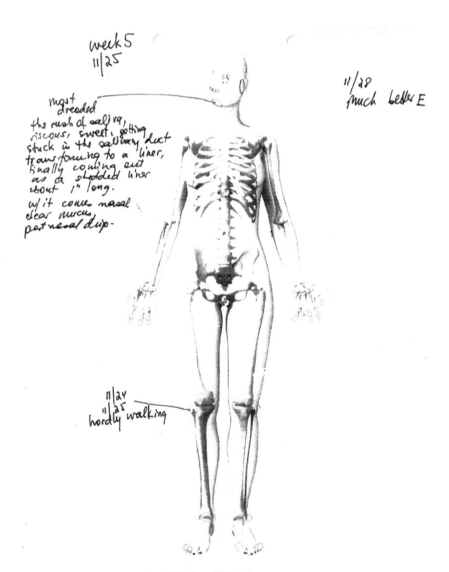

week 5
11/25

most
dreaded
the rush of saliva,
viscous, sweet, getting
stuck in the salivary duct
transforming to a liner,
finally coming out
as a shredded liner
about 1" long.
w/ it comes nasal
clear mucus,
post nasal drip-

11/28
much better E

11/24
11/25
hardly walking

While off Tindamax

Can Lyme disease induce allergic reactions?

Yes. More recently, there are articles emphasizing this is seen only in *Bartonella*, but the potential of Lyme to induce allergies has been discussed for thirty years. The hypothesis is based upon a non-specific stimulation of multiple components of the immune system including the part that is responsible for allergic reactions. Long before we recognized *Bartonella* as a coinfection, we knew that Lyme can be associated with new allergies. These allergic reactions usually subside when Lyme is successfully treated, but some people are left with persistent allergic tendencies. A similar presentation is described in CFS/ME called multiple chemical sensitivity syndrome.

One important allergy is the alpha-gal allergy. This is an allergy to red meats (e.g., beef, lamb) associated with the bite of a lone star tick. The scary part is that the allergic reaction occurs hours after eating it and often wakes people up with a severe allergic reaction, eight hours after eating beef for dinner. Tests are available to diagnose this. If positive, those individuals must avoid these meats.

I also need to address reactions to gluten in general and in this population in particular. Wheat has been genetically modified in the US, so there is an enhanced potential to "reject" it. This can be tested in so many different ways: gene testing to look for genetic predisposition, blood tests for IgA and IgG, stool tests for IgA, and the standard "celiac panel." Please do not make the error of thinking you cannot eat wheat/gluten *only* if you have a positive celiac panel. Any of the other antibody tests are suggesting that your immune system is reacting. IgA is made in the gut, and IgG is made in the blood. They are both important.

People with gut symptoms need to get good tests for allergies to food. This is different. It is an IgE test. Many times you will not find the offender, so keep good food journals, and find a common thread. There may be an eight-to-twelve-hour delay between eating the food and the reaction.

Treatment

For early cases, Doxycycline or Zithromax/Biaxin (macrolides) are effective. As I mentioned above, I give 6 weeks and in my practice, I add Tindamax in the 6th week to avoid the issue of round body formation. In my opinion, old studies stating that 90% of patients with early infections are "cured" with short courses of antibiotics are flawed. The follow up was inadequate. Adding Tindamax in the 6th week would totally eradicate any round bodies.

For late cases, more aggressive treatment is required. If the Cephalosporin group is used at all it cannot be given orally. In my retrospective study of 160 patients, as well as my overwhelming observation of patients treated with these drugs, they are ineffective unless IV Rocephin is added to an oral regimen. When cells infected with Borrelia are incubated with Rocephin (which applies to all Cephalosporins), it has no intracellular penetration. In humans, it is highly effective in the brain and does enter the joints, but it must be combined with an oral antibiotic that has good intracellular penetration. Minocycline has the highest brain penetration of the tetracycline group and is effective for arthritis. It also has other beneficial properties in the brain. Doxycycline has excellent joint penetration and is second to Minocycline for brain penetration. It also acts as an anti-inflammatory agent in joints and is approved for Rheumatoid Arthritis. All tetracyclines induce extreme sun sensitivity rashes, especially if combined with Celebrex which is often used in arthritis. Tindamax must always be added in some fashion. As I mentioned, I add it one week a month. If this is not tolerated, it is added 2 days a week.

Although Rifampin was recently found to be effective against persisters, I do not add it when a patient only has Lyme disease due to potential toxicity issues. Rifampin also interacts with many other medications.

Recent studies show Diflucan to be effective. Again, this is not added in my practice unless the patient has yeast overgrowth, or if they are not adequately responsive to all other modalities. Although studies in females with chronic yeast infections do show safety if used for 3 months, it can affect adrenal function. If added, I would add only 10 days a month. As mentioned, since the organism is unique, this type of treatment is acceptable. It has been used as an adjunct to treatment in Europe for many years. Other IV modalities are discussed in the Bartonella treatment section.

Patients must keep strict daily records and bring them in to appointments. I prefer a numerical system from 1-10 set in a spreadsheet with only relevant symptoms listed. The addition of Tindamax, or any other agent used intermittently must be listed for those days. For menstruating females, they must note their menstrual cycle. Symptoms are definitely affected by hormonal fluctuations. The relationship between hormonal changes and immunity has been studied in lupus patients.

Never rely on memory if you are a patient. Studies show that we are unable to accurately recollect past events, or even very recent events. Young people with cameras on their heads were unable to accurately report scenes they had just seen in a controlled setting. How on earth can a patient with short term memory loss, almost universal in most of these patients, be expected to retain that information? Also, people tend to report how they have felt in the past month with a huge bias based upon how they feel THAT day (the day of the office visit). It is common for a patient to report they feel "awful", but on review of their symptom sheets, they had a significant improvement over the past month, compared with the prior months.

The patient who graphically fills in affected joints, also makes detailed notes about all symptoms. She can see how dramatically worse she is on Tindamax, and how much she has improved over time. This is a vital tool. Doctors need to take the time to review these data (yes, data is a plural and used incorrectly in language all the time!). Doctors who rely on Insurance reimbursement cannot afford to take the time due to inadequate payments. Apparently our time is not valuable to insurance companies. That is sad given that the syndromes I mention in this book require arduous review of symptoms, blood tests, side effects and mandates a thorough physical examination at each and every visit to assess all of the manifestations that were abnormal in the past. I fully examine each patient at every appointment, and look at tongues and culture tongues that look like there is yeast overgrowth.

All patients must take refrigerated acidophilus with multiple strains at least 3 or more hours after the last antibiotic, usually at bedtime. They must take as many as is required to maintain normal bowel movements. Probiotics will not work because they are spores that turn into live gut bacteria in the gut. If an antibiotic is in the gut, it will kill most of the bacteria creating dysbiosis. This is dangerous. Saccharomyces survive antibiotics. It is strange that many doctors think that replacing only this bacterium is a good idea. It makes no sense. It already creates dysbiosis. All the other healthy gut bacteria need to be replenished if the gut is to survive antibiotics. All refined carbohydrates, additives, preservatives and pesticides MUST be avoided.

Role of Vitamin D in the immune system

2 5D is inactive and is converted to 1,25D which is active. One of the functions of 1,25D is to bind to something called the "VDR" (Vitamin D receptor) which is crucial to good immune function. Bacteria can bind to this receptor, thus downregulating immune function. One of the most important tests to look at is both the 25D level and the 1,5D level. A low 25D alone is viewed as an indicator of abnormal immune function. Many physicians test only the 25D and prescribe 1,25D (D3). This can be catastrophic in Lyme disease because it has a very high affinity for the VDR and often either the 1,25D is elevated or the ratio of 1,25D/25D is elevated. In this case, calcium is removed from bones and can cause osteoporosis. Although this is counter intuitive, it is an inflammatory reaction. Please make sure you measure both, even if some insurance companies have jointly decided not to reimburse for it.

Summary

As can be seen from the above, treatment of this complex infection is multifactorial and not simple. There is no *one* right answer! Each person must be assessed on the basis of their specific clinical presentation, taking into account the duration of untreated infection and other infections that need to be addressed, including both other tick-borne infections but also opportunistic infections that take advantage of immunosuppressed hosts such as EBV, CMV, Mycoplasma, HHV6, HSV1 and 2, and others.

The trivialization of Lyme disease by many in the medical community, with the tacit approval by the "leaders" in the field such as the IDSA and the CDC, has greatly hampered the education of doctors and the ability of those of us who are knowledgeable in this field to treat our patients to the best of our ability. In light of all the great research advances, this must stop. It is demeaning to educated physicians and restricts coverage for medically necessary treatment by insurance carriers. It is no coincidence that the "experts" hired by insurance carriers are selected from the IDSA and others who participate in the denial of all of the above-mentioned research that proves how complex these infections are.

To date, there are now fifty-four new species of *Borrelia*. The original organism identified as a cause of Lyme disease is *Borrelia burgdorferi*. Testing by most commercial laboratories are aimed at *only B. burgdorferi*. Isn't it obvious why so many infected people test negative?

1. *Borrelia afzelii* (Canica et al. 1994)
2. *Borrelia americana* (Rudenko et al. 2010)

3. *Borrelia andersonii* (Marconi et al. 1995)
4. *Borrelia anserina* (Sakharoff 1891; Bergey et al. 1925)
5. *Borrelia baltazardii* (ex Karimi et al. 1979; Karimi et al. 1983)
6. *Borrelia bavariensis* (Margos et al. 2009)
7. *Borrelia bissettii* (Postic et al. 1998)
8. *Borrelia brasiliensis* (Davis 1952)
9. *Borrelia burgdorferi* (Johnson et al. 1984 emend; Baranton et al. 1992 [Lyme disease spirochete])
10. *Borrelia californiensis* (Postic et al. 2007)
11. *Borrelia carolinensis* (Rudenko et al. 2011)
12. *Borrelia caucasica* (Kandelaki 1945; Davis 1957)
13. *Borrelia chilensis* (Ivanova et al. 2014)
14. *Borrelia coriaceae* (Johnson et al. 1987)
15. *Borrelia crocidurae* (Leger 1917; Davis 1957)
16. *Borrelia dugesii* (Mazzotti 1949; Davis 1957)
17. *Borrelia duttonii* (Novy and Knapp 1906; Bergey et al. 1925)
18. *Candidatus Borrelia finlandensis* (Casjens et al. 2011)
19. *Borrelia garinii* (Baranton et al. 1992)
20. *Borrelia graingeri* (Heisch 1953; Davis 1957)
21. *Borrelia harveyi* (Garnham 1947; Davis 1948)
22. *Borrelia hermsii* (Davis 1942; Steinhaus 1946)
23. *Borrelia hispanica* (de Buen 1926; Steinhaus 1946)
24. *Borrelia japonica* (Kawabata et al. 1994)
25. *Candidatus Borrelia johnsonii* (Schwan et al. 2009)
26. *Candidatus Borrelia kalaharica* (Fingerle et al. 2016)
27. *Borrelia kurtenbachii* (Margos et al. 2010)
28. *Borrelia latyschewii* (Sofiev 1941; Davis 1948)
29. *Borrelia lonestari* (Barbour et al. 1996)
30. *Borrelia lusitaniae* (Le Fleche et al. 1997)
31. *Borrelia mayonii* (Pritt et al. 2016)
32. *Borrelia mazzottii* (Davis 1956)
33. *Borrelia merionesi* (Hougen 1974)
34. *Borrelia microti*

35. *Borrelia miyamotoi* (Fukunaga et al. 1995)
36. *Candidatus Borrelia mvumii* (Mitani et al. 2014)
37. *Borrelia parkeri* (Davis 1942; Steinhaus 1946)
38. *Borrelia persica* (Dschunkowsky 1913; Steinhaus 1946)
39. *Borrelia queenslandica* (PopeJG et al. 1962)
40. *Borrelia recurrentis* (Lebert 1874; Bergey et al. 1925)
41. *Borrelia sinica* (Masuzawa et al. 2001)
42. *Borrelia spielmanii* (Richter et al. 2006)
43. *Candidatus Borrelia tachyglossi* (Loh et al. 2016)
44. *Borrelia tanukii* (Fukunaga et al. 1997)
45. *Candidatus Borrelia texasensis* (Lin et al. 2005)
46. *Borrelia theileri* (Laveran 1903; Bergey et al. 1925)
47. *Borrelia tillae* (Zumpt and Organ 1961)
48. *Borrelia turcica* (Güner et al. 2004)
49. *Borrelia turdi* (Fukunaga et al. 1997)
50. *Borrelia turicatae* (Brumpt 1933; Steinhaus 1946)
51. *Borrelia valaisiana* (Wang et al. 1997)
52. *Borrelia venezuelensis* (Brumpt 1921; Brumpt 1922)
53. *Borrelia vincentii*
54. *Borrelia yangtzensis* (Margos et al. 2015)

Given this, it is no surprise that testing is inadequate. Some test kits are better than others, but we are also hampered by the dogmatic assertion by the IDSA that you must be "CDC positive" to be diagnosed with Lyme. This is false. In fact, people with chronic neurological Lyme disease often lose antibodies as they become immunosuppressed. This is not unexpected since the organisms that cause Lyme and syphilis are very similar. It is well documented that when syphilis is advanced, those patients lose antibodies. It is also hampered by the fact that the CDC has omitted two very important antibodies on the Western Blot (31 and 34). In addition, almost every GP or "PCP" checks off the box that says, "ELISA with reflex to Western Blot." This is outdated and will miss even more cases. They *must* check the box that is looking at the Western Blot and the C6 Peptide Assay. This would enhance the diagnosis. In my thirty years, I rarely seen a doctor check off the C6 Peptide Assay. Interestingly the veterinarians are always more advanced than human doctors, and apparently they always do the C6 Peptide Assay on animals suspected of Lyme!

Bartonella

This is as prevalent in ticks as Lyme. MDL, a NJ-based company, funded a study looking at the prevalence of infections in ticks collected from different areas of the state. The prevalence of *B. burgdorferi* and *Bartonella henselae* was almost identical. The article is listed below.

Is Bartonella *more prevalent than Lyme?*

Bartonella is a much greater threat to humans than Lyme because it has been found to be carried by every animal tested in every country where testing has been performed. All animals appear to be hosts except for sea otters (they get endocarditis) and domesticated animals. In the past, it was called cat scratch disease because it was known to be found in 90 percent of feral cats. Most cats do not get sick from it, but some indoor cats manifest the infection. If you review old literature about this infection, it is trivialized because if it is transmitted by a cat scratch, it is usually self-limited. This is not the case when transmitted by an infected insect!

Which insects transmit Bartonella?

1. ticks
2. fleas
3. biting flies, including sand flies
4. lice
5. chiggers
6. mosquitoes

The species discussed most with regard to deer ticks is *Bartonella henselae*, but homeless people or others exposed to lice get *Bartonella quintana*. The presentation is different in the two species. There are other subspecies I will not cover here.

I wrote the first article on a patient who was found to have both *B. burgdorferi* plus *B. henselae* in both spinal fluid and blood. I recognized her rash as being that seen in cat scratch disease, thus prompting me to test her. By then, there was a study from the Netherlands in which *B. henselae* was found in their deer ticks. I presented her case plus other cases diagnosed around the same time. Those cases were published by Mordechai et al. My case report was ready to go to a journal, but the coauthor, who was a prominent infectious disease specialist in NJ, declined to put his name on the paper at the last minute. This is one of many examples of the censorship in this community. This man worked the case with me all along, because I thought he would be interested, and at the last minute, was not willing to threaten his "image" in the IDSA! There was no way I would get published without his name, and he knew it. It is very common for Lyme literate doctors (referred to as "LLMD's") to be unable to get articles published. There is a clear bias within mainstream clinical journals against publishing articles from physicians who treat chronic Lyme disease.

The pathophysiology of *Bartonella* is based upon two major presentations:

1. *Infection of endothelial cells.* These cells line all blood vessels. In endothelial cell cultures, the addition of live *Bartonella* bacteria results in replication of the cells and secretes an attractant that attracts the cells toward the bacteria. One marker that can be identified is VEGF, but other markers are being found by research in Germany. The result is thickening of these cells in capillaries, veins, and arteries. This causes hemangiomas in the skin and other organs, but more importantly, the arteries have a narrow lumen through which blood flows, thereby threatening oxygen

supply to the small blood vessels (fingers, toes, brain, deep muscles, nose, and patella). This results in severe cold intolerance, an internal feeling of "always feeling cold" despite external temperatures. Paradoxically the effect on capillaries is flushing of the skin, often magnified after a hot shower or bath.

I look for findings on physical examination that are strongly associated with *Bartonella* that differentiates it from Lyme.

Since every organ in the body depend upon oxygen delivery via arteries, it can affect multiple organ systems. The bacteria have "suction" cups that attach to heart valves, thus causing endocarditis. They can even attach to the outside of PICC lines or other indwelling devices. Marna Ericson found it on the outside of her son's PICC line when she saw a film on the PICC line as it was being removed.

2. *Red cells. Bartonella* goes into the blood and invades red cells intermittently and causes them to burst. This is subtle and does not cause what most hematologists think of as "acute hemolytic anemia." One hematologist mocked me recently, insisting that if a patient had hemolysis, they would have jaundice. This is not the case. The process is slow and intermittent. It is true that hemoglobin released from the cells is metabolized to bilirubin, but in many cases, one must review many blood tests to find the few with an elevated bilirubin. In the past, these cases were diagnosed with Gilbert syndrome, but now there is a test to confirm that diagnosis. When red cells are killed, the bone marrow must produce a higher number of red cells, which are called reticulocytes. These may or may not be elevated in chronic cases.

The presence of these bacteria in blood makes them accessible to the many insects that are now known to carry it and transmit it to humans. As we displace animals from their natural habitat, we will come into contact with the insects that bite them, and more infections will ensue.

I would say, based upon the ubiquitous nature of this bacterium and the difficulty getting a positive test, that is *very* likely that there are far more cases of *Bartonella* than Lyme. I would not be surprised if cases are misdiagnosed as "idiopathic" vasculitis, which means unknown origin.

Should diagnosis be based upon tests? No!

Other tests such as an elevated VEGF or elevated absolute reticulocyte counts can be helpful, as can the size of red cells called MCV. If you have *Bartonella*, the red cells are invaded roughly every five days. This results in death of the red cells (called hemolysis), so the bone marrow is forced to produce more "baby red cells" called reticulocytes. These are much larger than regular red cells, which live for six weeks in the blood. Thus, the average MCV will be high. In addition, the hemoglobin in the red cells is metabolized to bilirubin. This does not occur at a rapid rate, so the bilirubin may be only slightly elevated.

Bartonella is more likely than Lyme to result in elevated white cell counts, elevated sedimentation rates and elevated CRP levels. Lyme frequently does not act like a "typical" bacterial infection.

The tests are not accurate enough. If a person has ice-cold hands, feet, and nose; gets patches of red skin after hot baths; and has unexplained flushing; this infection should be suspected.

The fingers and toes as well as the kneecaps are ice-cold and often discolored. The palms get a mottled appearance. Each white area is an area of lack of blood flow, creating the "mottled" look. The palms are often blue toward the fingertips, and the veins are often more prominent.

The fingers are completely different from Raynaud's phenomenon. In the above, there is a distinct line below which the skin is purple or white due to arterial spasm. In *Bartonella*, the fingers and toes and the kneecaps are just purple with no distinct line and often even in a warm room. My examining room is kept at 70 degrees Fahrenheit when these photos were taken.

Bartonella rashes. Do they really look like cat scratches? Yes!

The marks you see on these numerous patients were not scratches and suddenly appeared. I ask people if they have cats or were outdoors in the woods. They are people who are inside and do not feel well enough to be outside.

The one rash is the type of flushing I see in *Bartonella*.

The other rash that looks like a type of acne is also a *Bartonella* rash.

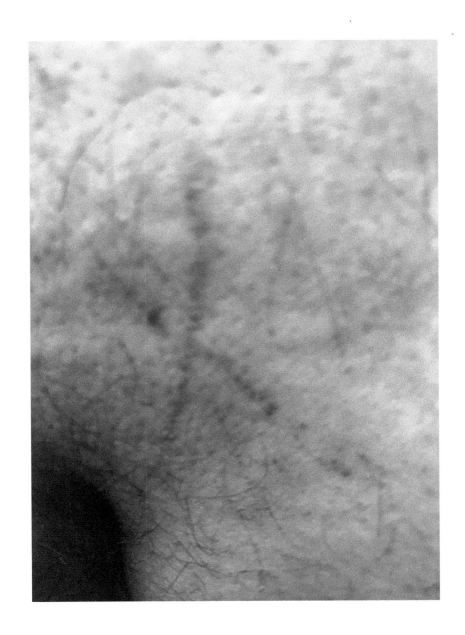

AM I CRAZY?

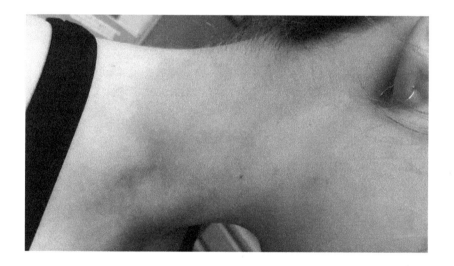

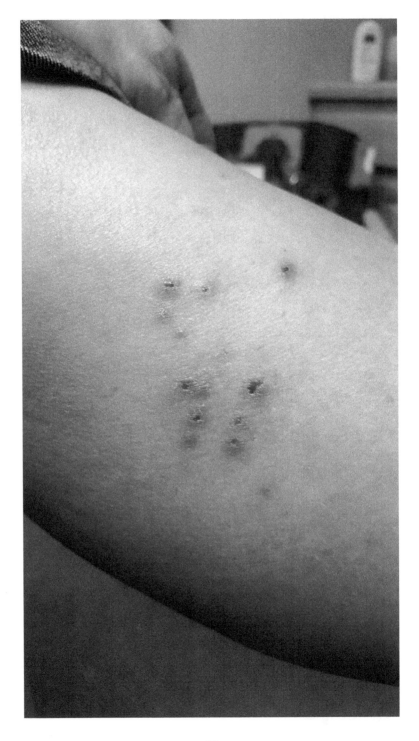

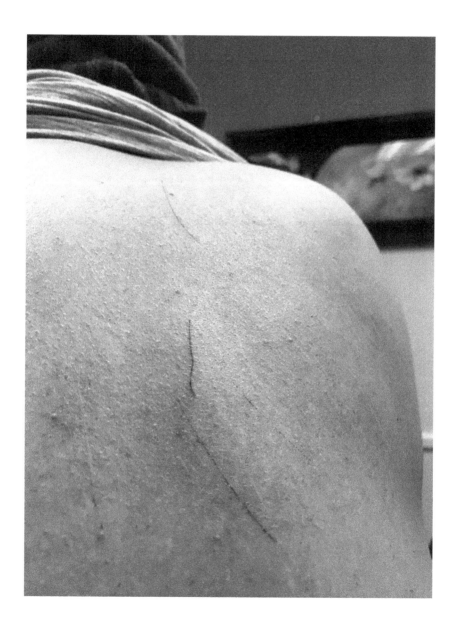

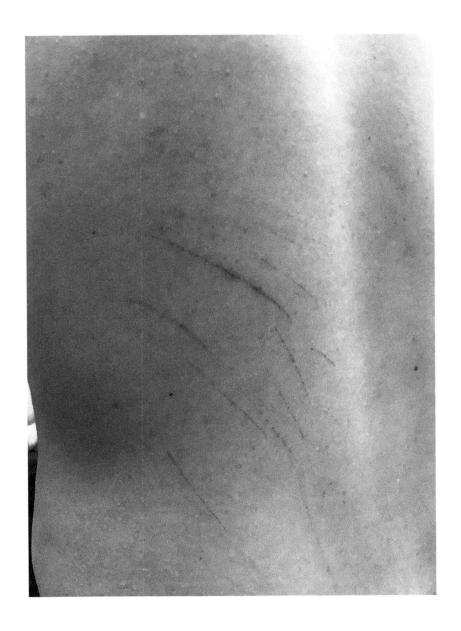

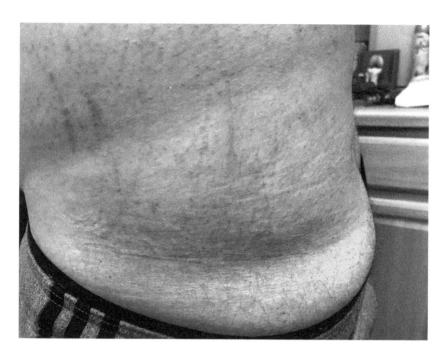

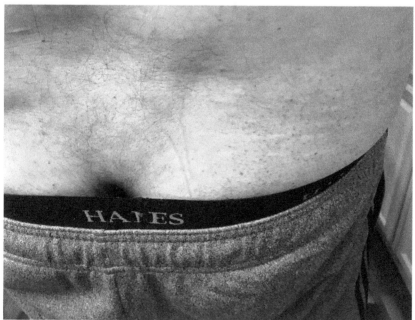

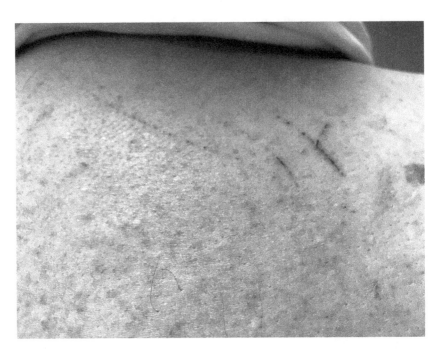

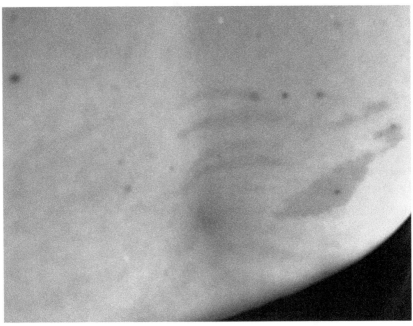

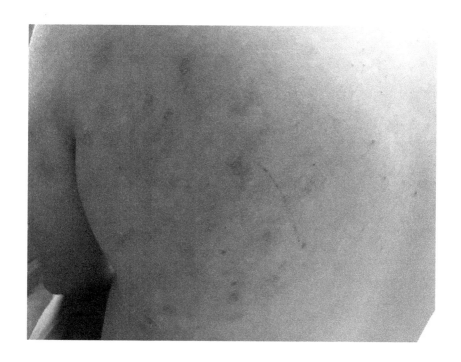

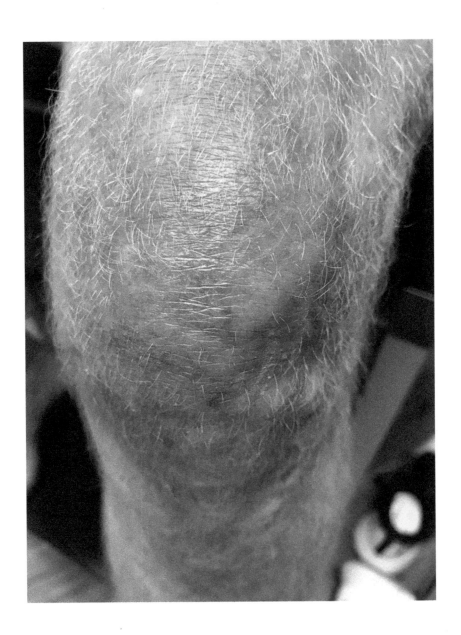

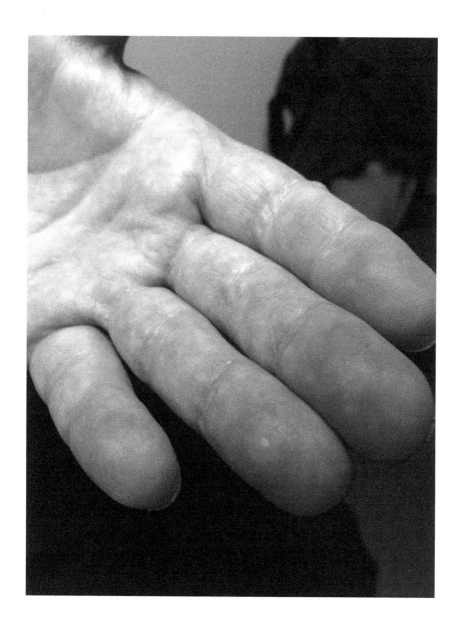

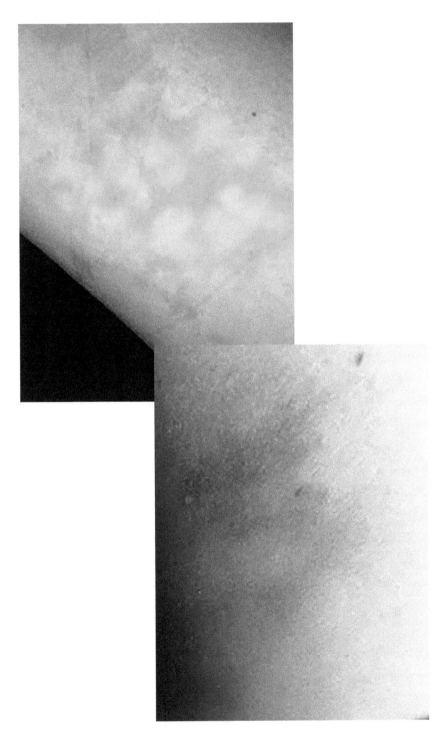

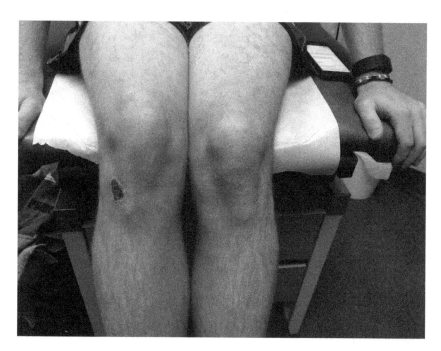

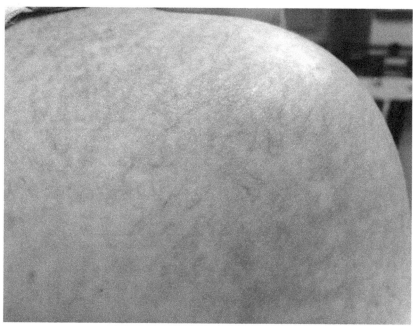

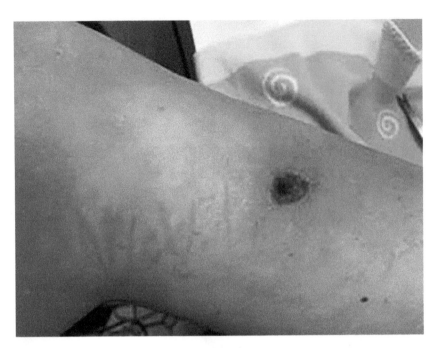

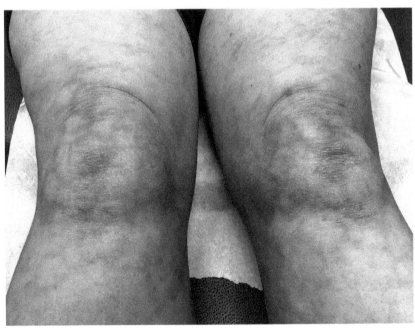

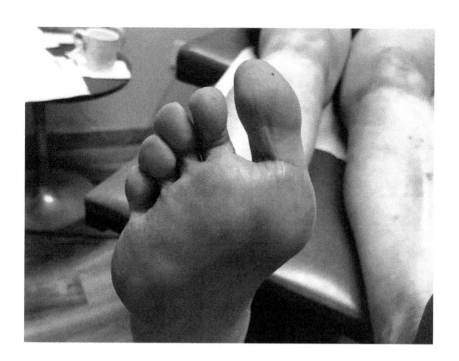

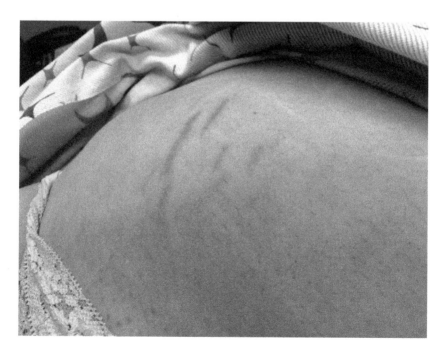

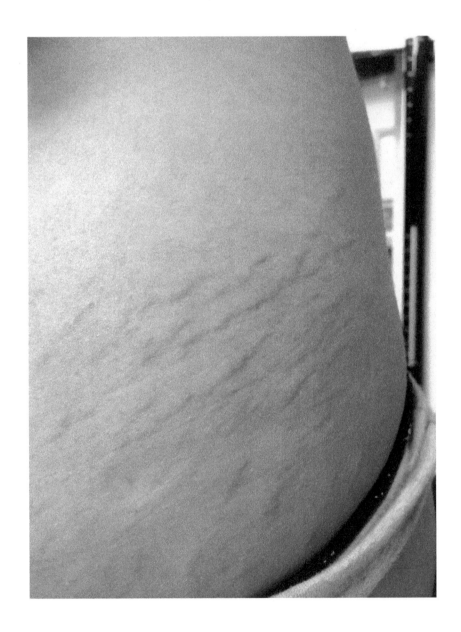

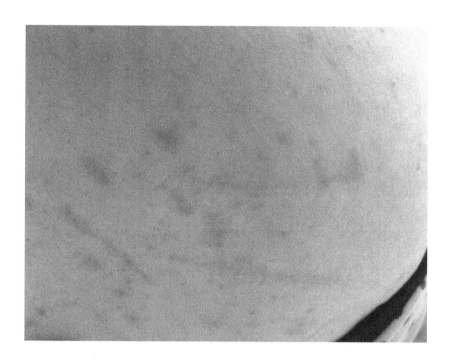

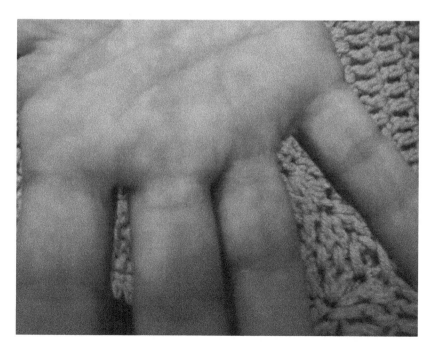

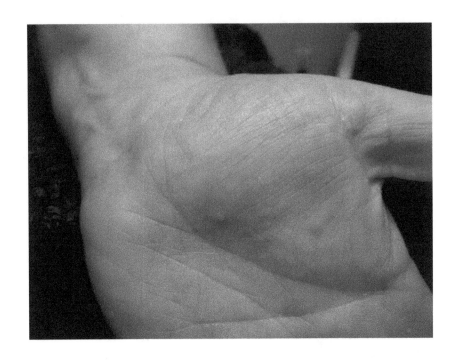

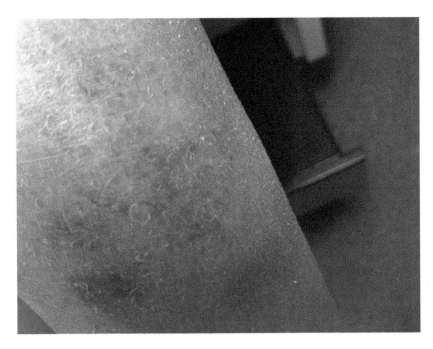

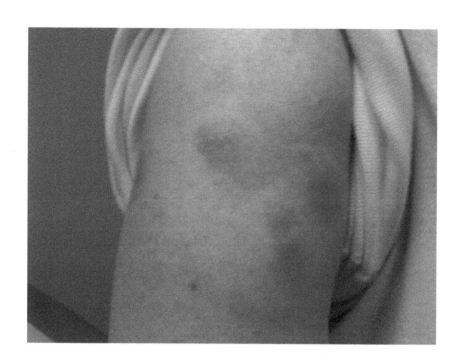

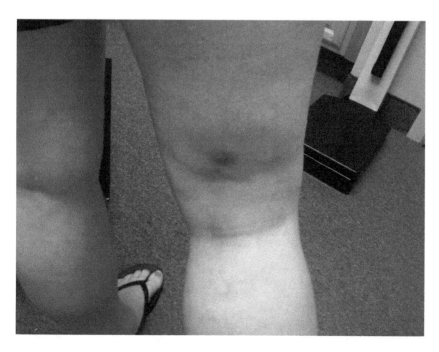

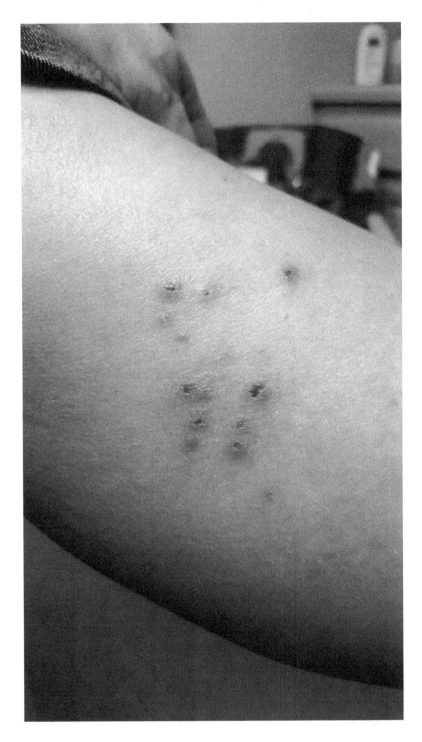

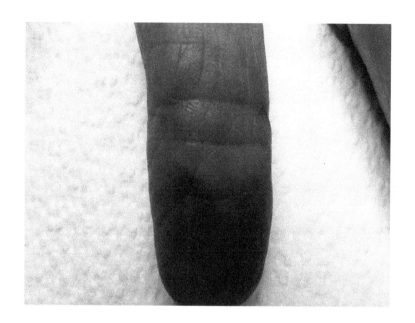

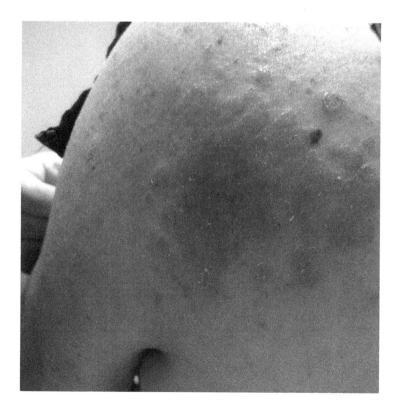

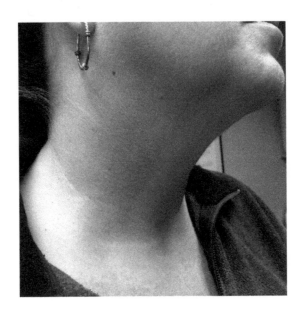

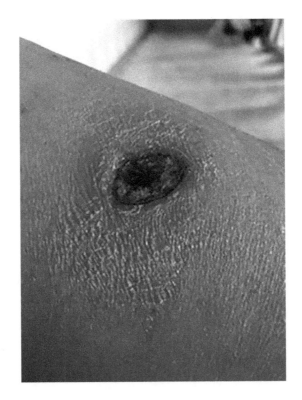

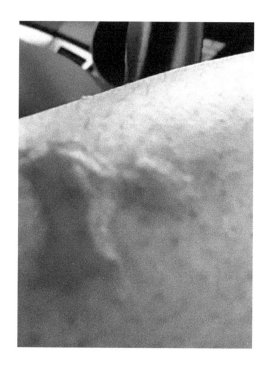

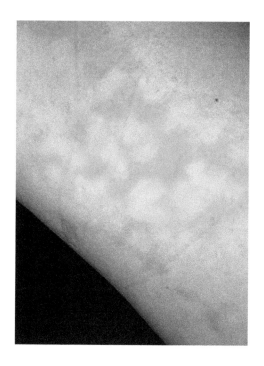

The clinical findings must be analyzed, and a decision must be made whether the history plus the examination adequately fulfills the diagnosis of *Bartonella*. This is especially relevant in someone exposed to multiple insect species: flies, mosquitoes, fleas, ticks, lice, etc.

In addition, the vibration sensation in extremities can be blunted because the nerves depend upon arteries for their nutrients.

This is one of the many reasons "remote" medicine, which is now being purported as an adequate replacement for a proper physical examination, is inadequate.

Microbiology of *Bartonella*

Most of the original and current research has been performed by the teams of Dr. Breitschwerdt in the USA, Dr. Kempf in Germany and Dr. Didier Raoult in France. The same researchers at John Hopkins University who demonstrated persister forms of Lyme have now also published articles about these forms in *Bartonella* species. As it turns out, many bacteria have persister forms that develop in response to antibiotics, and many also form biofilms. *Bartonella* has not been found under biofilms yet but most likely will be found to either manufacture them or live inside them, as has been found with other bacterial species. *Chlamydia pneumoniae* for example has been elegantly examined by Dr. Wilmore Webley (YouTube) who shows that multiple bacteria can exist under biofilms. Dr. Sapi published that *Borrelia* and *Chlamydia pneumoniae* exist under the same biofilm.

Despite this research, I think it is premature to initiate treatment based upon these "persister" studies because we do not know enough about these forms in humans. In addition, many of the substances shown to kill the persister forms are not even available in oral or IV form. I have listed the research papers for people who want to know more about these studies.

The reference section covers these studies.

Dental Manifestations in Lyme disease and Bartonella

Many patients with Lyme disease can present to dentists with either TMJ or unexplained dental pain. The TMJ is the fourth commonest joint involved in Lyme arthritis. I am affiliated with the TMJ Department at Rutgers as an adjunct faculty hoping to cover the importance of this. In addition, patients with Lyme can experience referred pain in their mouth and teeth that is based upon neuropathies. This means that the teeth are fine but the pain is a manifestation of nerve inflammation. Dr. Gary Heir (Clinical Professor, Director Division of Orofacial Pain, American Academy of Orofacial Pain, American Association for Study of Headache, American Board of Orofacial Pain, American Dental Association, Association of Migraine Disorders, ICOT-International Congress of Orofacial Pain and Temporomandibular Disorders, International Association for the Study of Pain, International Headache Society) and I published several articles in dental journals listed in the reference section about the dangers of potentially unnecessary invasive dental procedures in these patients.

Bartonella, on the other hand, can cause severe gingivitis and I have had two young females lose their teeth due to severe bone erosion in their jaws. Cats with dental disease as a result of bartonella have severe gingivitis and dental decay. I have observed a nasty film on the tongues of many patients with Bartonella with repeatedly negative cultures for yeast.

There are two publications where a 2,000 year old tooth and a 4,000 year old tooth had positive Bartonella PCR's in the pulp. This further confirms a strong relationship between dental decay and this organism.

Since the upper teeth are close to the maxillary sinuses, it can invade sinuses where it finds a comfortable niche to remain. It is now possible to send cultures for Bartonella to Galaxy Laboratory in North Carolina. They are not testing teeth, but if fluid from sinuses is drained, they could culture that, as well as blood samples.

Treatment

In my opinion, there is no recipe I can give anyone to treat a specific patient. Many patients have more than one pathogen to deal with and have developed either ME or FM or both.

Dr. Breitschwerdt is adamant that this bacterium will become resistant to Zithromax very quickly, so I avoid this antibiotic. The common understanding based upon *in vitro* research is that combinations need to be used. The most common is doxycycline or minocycline plus rifampin or Bactrim/Septra. The Quinolone group (Cipro, Levaquine etc.) is effective in both the older studies and recent ones regarding the persisters, but the chronic use of these medications have unacceptably high potential side effects. Gentamycin is highly effective for both the common forms and the persisters. If a patient is on intravenous antibiotics, this is a potent and effective treatment. Peak and trough levels need to be done although I have found that 5 days a week is safe and effective. In that setting the trough can still be done but I have not seen any side effects to date. Vancomycin was found by Raoult to be universally effective in his studies, however Breitschwerdt cannot say the same. It is also a good choice if a patient is on IV, especially is they also have Lyme disease because there is a very compelling study showing how effective this is against Borrelia, and if weekly IM BiCillin is added, the study showed incredible synergism between the two in Lyme. Once again, if you stick to 4-5 days a week, it is not necessary to perform peak and trough levels.

The only studies in humans are those relating to HIV patients who succumb to *Bartonella*. There are no good studies yet on insect-transmitted *Bartonella* in previously healthy people.

Studies addressing the stationary phase of Bartonella include other modalities such as methylene blue. Please keep in mind that these are petri-dish studies, and there is no data on the long-term use of this agent.

In general, I believe that diet and supplements as well as adequate rest and lack of stress are even more important than antibiotics. If you are so stressed and sleep-deprived that your immune system is functioning at a low level, no antibiotics on earth are going to work. Several studies elegantly demonstrate that as stress increases, immune function decreases in a linear fashion. You need an intact immune system to combat these pathogens if you have any chance of beating these diseases. The main areas of immune control are the brain and the gut.

The government has been punishing doctors who prescribe pain medications. How can someone in chronic pain ever get better if we do not treat the pain? As mentioned earlier, chronic pain induces fibromyalgia. We cannot prevent this if we refuse to treat the pain. I am not suggesting that everyone should be given narcotics, but if they have failed gabapentin, Lyrica, non-addicting sleep medications, acupuncture, cupping, and other modalities and continue to have pain or lack of restorative sleep, then as doctors, we need to step up to the plate and treat our patients to the best of our ability.

In summary, as doctors, we need to look at each patient as a whole and treat every component instead of writing a prescription for three weeks of doxycycline and sit back thinking the patient has been adequately treated!

As patients, you need to educate yourselves and be advocates for your medical care. This is the unfortunate truth. You will not get better if you do not consider the role of sleep, diet, and stress. Do not trivialize the importance of these frequently overlooked issues.

I hope this short book is read by both doctors and patients alike so that this message is received.

I blame insurance companies for their pathetic reimbursement for a doctor's time and for the breakdown in medicine today. A physician cannot afford to take the time required to treat complicated patients because they would be bankrupt. That is a whole different book!

For patients out there suffering, *you are not crazy!*

References

Adelson, Martin E., Raja-Venkitesh S. Rao, Richard C. Tilton, Kimberly Cabets, Eugene Eskow, Lesley Fein, James L. Occi, and Eli Mordechai. 2004. "Prevalence of *Borrelia burgdorferi, Bartonella* spp., *Babesia microti,* and *Anaplasma phagocytophila* in *Ixodes scapularis* Ticks Collected in Northern New Jersey." *Journal of Clinical Microbiology* 42, no. 6 (June). https://doi.org/10.1128/JCM.42.6.2799-2801.2004.

Aucott, John N. 2015. "Posttreatment Lyme Disease Syndrome." *Infectious Disease Clinics of North America* 29, no. 2 (June): 309–323. https://doi.org/10.1016/j.idc.2015.02.012.

Baker, Phillip J. 2008. "Beating Lyme: *Understanding and treating this complex and often misdiagnosed disease.*" *The Journal of Clinical Investigation* 118, no. 9 (September 2): 2,990. https://doi.org/10.1172/JCI36641.

Balakrishnan, Nandhakumar, Marna Ericson, Ricardo Maggi, and Edward B. Breitschwerdt. 2016. "Vasculitis, Cerebral Infarction and Persistent *Bartonella henselae* Infection in a Child." *Parasites & Vectors* 9, article no. 254. https://doi.org/10.1186/s13071-016-1547-9.

BHA Mai, R Barbieri, T Chenal, D Castex, R Jonvel…—PloS one, 2020—journals.plos.org. [HTML] Five millennia of *Bartonella quintana* bacteraemia.

Blum, Lisa K., Julia Z. Adamska, Dale S. Martin, Alison W. Rebman, Serra E. Elliott, Richard R. L. Cao, Monica E. Embers, John N. Aucott, Mark J. Soloski, and William H. Robinson. 2018. "Robust B Cell Responses Predict Rapid Resolution of Lyme

Disease." *Frontiers in Immunology* 9 (July 18), article no. 1634. https://doi.org/10.3389/fimmu.2018.01634.

Bransfield, Robert C. 2018. "Neuropsychiatric Lyme Borreliosis: An Overview with a Focus on a Specialty Psychiatrist's Clinical Practice." *Healthcare* 6, no. 3: 104. https://doi.org/10.3390/healthcare6030104.

Breitschwerdt, Edward Bealmear. 2014. "Bartonellosis: One Health Perspectives for an Emerging Infectious Disease." *ILAR Journal* 55, no. 1:46–58. https://doi.org/10.1093/ilar/ilu015.

Breitschwerdt, E. B., K. L. Linder, M. J. Day, R. G. Maggi, B. B. Chomel, V. A. J. Kempf. 2013. "Koch's Postulates and the Pathogenesis of Comparative Infectious Disease Causation Associated with *Bartonella* Species." *Journal of Comparative Pathology* 148, no. 2–3: 115–125. https://doi.org/10.1016/j.jcpa.2012.12.003.

Breitschwerdt, E. B., S. Sontakke, and S. Hopkins. 2012. "Neurological Manifestations of Bartonellosis in Immunocompetent Patients: A Composite of Reports from 2005–2012." *Journal of Neuroparasitology* 3, article ID 235640. https://doi.org/10.4303/jnp/235640.

Breitschwerdt, Edward B., Patricia E. Mascarelli, Lori A. Schweickert, Ricardo G. Maggi, Barbara C. Hegarty, Julie M. Bradley, and Christopher W. Woods. 2011. "Hallucinations, Sensory Neuropathy, and Peripheral Visual Deficits in a Young Woman Infected with *Bartonella koehlerae*." *Journal of Clinical Microbiology* 49, no. 9 (August 30). https://doi.org/10.1128/JCM.00833-11.

Breitschwerdt, Edward B., Ricardo G. Maggi, Maria Belen Cadenas, and Pedro Paulo Vissotto de Paiva Diniz. 2009. "A Groundhog, a Novel *Bartonella* Sequence, and My Father's Death." *Emerging Infectious Diseases* 15, no. 12 (December): 2,080–2,086. https://doi.org/10.3201/eid1512.090206.

Breitschwerdt, E. B., R. G. Maggi, W. L. Nicholson, N. A. Cherry, and C. W. Woods. 2008. "*Bartonella* sp. Bacteremia in Patients with Neurological and Neurocognitive Dysfunction." *Journal of Clinical Microbiology* 46, no. 9 (September). https://doi.org/10.1128/JCM.00832-08.

Breitschwerdt, Edward B., Ricardo G. Maggi, Ashlee W. Duncan, William L. Nicholson, Barbara C. Hegarty, and Christopher W. Woods. 2007. "*Bartonella* Species in Blood of Immunocompetent Persons with Animal and Arthropod Contact." *Emerging Infectious Diseases* 13, no. 6 (June): 938–941. https://doi.org/10.3201/eid1306.061337.

Coughlin, Jennifer M., Ting Yang, Alison W. Rebman, Kathleen T. Bechtold, Yong Du, William B. Mathews, Wojciech G. Lesniak, Erica A. Mihm, Sarah M. Frey, Erica S. Marshall, Hailey B. Rosenthal, Tristan A. Reekie, Michael Kassiou, Robert F. Dannals, Mark J. Soloski, John N. Aucott, and Martin G. Pomper. 2018. "Imaging Glial Activation in Patients with Post-Treatment Lyme Disease Symptoms: a Pilot Study Using [^{11}C]DPA-713 PET." *Journal of Neuroinflammation* 15, article no. 346 (December 19). https://doi.org/10.1186/s12974-018-1381-4.

Coulter, Peggy, Clara Lema, Diane Flayhart, Amy S. Linhardt, John N. Aucott, Paul G. Auwaerter, and J. Stephen Dumler. 2005. "Two-Year Evaluation of *Borrelia burgdorferi* Culture and Supplemental Tests for Definitive Diagnosis of Lyme Disease." *Journal of Clinical Microbiology* 43, no. 10 (October). https://doi.org/10.1128/JCM.43.10.5080-5084.2005.

Dever, Lisa, James H. Jorgensen and Alan G. Barbour. In Vitro Activity of Vancomycin against Spirochete Borrelia burgdorferi. Antimicrobial Agents and Chemotherapy, May 1993, pages 1115-1121

Dietrich, Florian, Thomas Schmidgen, Ricardo G. Maggi, Dania Richter, Franz-Rainer Matuschka, Reinhard Vonthein, Edward B. Breitschwerdt, and Volkhard A. J. Kempf. 2010. "Prevalence of *Bartonella henselae* and *Borrelia burgdorferi* Sensu Lato DNA in *Ixodes ricinus* Ticks in Europe." *Applied and Environmental Microbiology* 76, no. 5 (January 8). https://doi.org/10.1128/AEM.02788-09.

Diniz, Pedro Paulo Vissotto de Paiva, Paulo Eduardo Neves Ferreira Velho, Luiza Helena Urso Pitassi, Marina Rovani Drummond, Bruno Grosselli Lania, Maria Lourdes Barjas-Castro, Stanley Sowy, Edward B. Breitschwerdt, and Diana Gerardi Scorpio. 2016. "Risk Factors for *Bartonella* Species Infection in Blood Donors from Southeast Brazil." *PLOS Neglected Tropical Diseases* (March 21). https://doi.org/10.1371/journal.pntd.0004509.

Duncan, Ashlee W., Ricardo G. Maggi, and Edward B. Breitschwerdt. 2007. "*Bartonella* DNA in Dog Saliva." *Emerging Infectious Diseases* 13, no. 12 (December): 1,948–1,950. https://doi.org/10.3201/eid1312.070653.

Fallon, Brian A., Felice Tager, John Keilp, Nicola Weiss, Michael R. Liebowitz, Lesley Fein, and Kenneth Liegner. 1999. "Repeated Antibiotic Treatment in Chronic Lyme Disease." *Journal of Spirochetal and Tick-Borne Diseases* 6, no. 4: 94–102. http://www.lymeeducation.com/reference_documents/Repeated%20Antibiotic%20Treatment%20in%20Chronic%20Lyme%20Disease.pdf

Feng, Jie, Tingting Li, Rebecca Yee, Yuting Yuan, Chunxiang Bai, Menghua Cai, Wanliang Shi, Monica Embers, Cory Brayton, Harumi Saeki, Kathleen Gabrielson, Ying Zhang. 2019. "Stationary Phase Persister/Biofilm Microcolony of *Borrelia burgdorferi* Causes More Severe Disease in a Mouse Model of Lyme Arthritis: Implications for Understanding Persistence, Post-Treatment Lyme Disease Syndrome (PTLDS), and Treatment Failure." *Discovery Medicine* 27, no. 148 (March): 125–138. https://www.discoverymedicine.com/Jie-Feng/2019/03/persister-biofilm-microcolony-borrelia-burg-dorferi-causes-severe-lyme-arthritis-in-mouse-model.

Feng, Jie, Wanliang Shi, Shuo Zhang, David Sullivan, Paul G. Auwaerter, and Ying Zhang. 2016. "A Drug Combination Screen Identifies Drugs Active against Amoxicillin-Induced Round Bodies of *In Vitro Borrelia burgdorferi* Persisters from an FDA Drug Library." *Frontiers in Microbiology* (May 23). https://doi.org/10.3389/fmicb.2016.00743.

Feng, Jie, Shuo Zhang, Wanliang Shi, and Ying Zhang. 2016. "Ceftriaxone Pulse Dosing Fails to Eradicate Biofilm-Like Microcolony *B. burgdorferi* Persisters Which Are Sterilized by Daptomycin/ Doxycycline/Cefuroxime without Pulse Dosing." *Frontiers in Microbiology* 7 (November 4), article no. 1744. https://doi.org/10.3389/fmicb.2016.01744.

Feng, Jie, Wanliang Shi, Shuo Zhang, and Ying Zhang. 2015. "Persister Mechanisms in *Borrelia burgdorferi*: Implications for Improved Intervention." *Emerging Microbes & Infections* 4, no. 1. https://doi.org/10.1038/emi.2015.51.

Feng, Jie, Megan Weitner, Wanliang Shi, Shuo Zhang, David Sullivan, and Ying Zhang. 2015. "Identification of Additional Anti-Persister Activity against *Borrelia burgdorferi* from an FDA Drug Library." *Antibiotics* 4, no. 3: 397–410. https://doi.org/10.3390/antibiotics4030397.

Feng, Jie, Paul G. Auwaerter, Ying Zhang. 2015. "Drug Combinations against *Borrelia burgdorferi* Persisters *In Vitro*: Eradication Achieved by Using Daptomycin, Cefoperazone, and Doxycycline." *PLOS ONE* (March 25). https://doi.org/10.1371/journal.pone.0117207.

Feng, Jie, Wanliang Shi, Shuo Zhang, and Ying Zhang. 2015. "Identification of New Compounds with High Activity against Stationary Phase *Borrelia burgdorferi* from the NCI Compound Collection." *Emerging Microbes & Infections* 4, no. 1 (January 25). https://doi.org/10.1038/emi.2015.31.

Feng, Jie, Ting Wang, Wanliang Shi, Shuo Zhang, David Sullivan, Paul G. Auwaerter, and Ying Zhang. 2014. "Identification of Novel Activity against *Borrelia burgdorferi* Persisters Using an FDA-Approved Drug Library." *Emerging Microbes & Infections* 3, no. 1. https://doi.org/10.1038/emi.2014.53.

Fülöp, Tamàs, Ruth F. Itzhaki, Brian J. Balin, Judith Miklossy, and Annelise E. Barron. 2018. "Role of Microbes in the Development of Alzheimer's Disease: State of the Art—An International Symposium Presented at the 2017 IAGG Congress in San

Francisco." *Frontiers in Genetics* 9 (September 10), article no. 362. https://doi.org/10.3389/fgene.2018.00362.

Heir, Gary M., and Lesley A. Fein. 1996. "Lyme Disease: Considerations for Dentistry." *Journal of Orofacial Pain* 10, no. 1: 74–86. http://www.quintpub.com/userhome/jop/jop_10_1_heir_10.pdf.

Kaisera, Patrick O., Tanja Riess, Fiona O'Rourke, Dirk Linke, and Volkhard A. J. Kempfa. 2011. "*Bartonella* spp.: Throwing Light on Uncommon Human Infections." *International Journal of Medical Microbiology* 301, no. 1 (January): 7–15. https://doi.org/10.1016/j.ijmm.2010.06.004.

Karem, Kevin L., Christopher D. Paddock, and Russell L. Regnery. 2000. "*Bartonella henselae, B. quintana*, and *B. bacilliformis*: Historical Pathogens of Emerging Significance." *Microbes and Infection* 2, no. 10 (August): 1,193–1,205. https://doi.org/10.1016/S1286-4579(00)01273-9.

Kempf, Volkhard A. J., Bettina Volkmann, Martin Schaller, Christian A. Sander, Kari Alitalo, Tanja Rieß, Ingo B. Autenrieth. 2001. "Evidence of a Leading Role for VEGF in *Bartonella henselae*-Induced Endothelial Cell Proliferations." *Cellular Microbiology* 3, no. 9 (September): 623–632. https://doi.org/10.1046/j.1462-5822.2001.00144.x.

Kempf, V. A. J., M. Schaller, S. Behrendt, B. Volkmann, M. Aepfelbacher, I. Cakman, and I. B. Autenrieth. 2000. "Interaction of *Bartonella henselae* with Endothelial Cells Results in Rapid Bacterial rRNA Synthesis and Replication." *Cellular Microbiology* 2, no. 5 (October): 431–441. https://doi.org/10.1046/j.1462-5822.2000.00072.x.

MacDonald, Alan B. 2006. "Plaques of Alzheimer's Disease Originate from Cysts of *Borrelia burgdorferi*, the Lyme Disease Spirochete." *Medical Hypotheses* 67, no. 3: 592–600. https://doi.org/10.1016/j.mehy.2006.02.035.

Maggi, Ricardo G., B. Robert Mozayeni, Elizabeth L. Pultorak, Barbara C. Hegarty, Julie M. Bradley, Maria Correa, and Edward B. Breitschwerdt. 2012. "*Bartonella* spp. Bacteremia and Rheumatic Symptoms in Patients from Lyme Disease—Endemic Region." *Emerging Infectious Diseases* 18, no. 5 (May): 783–791. https://doi.org/10.3201/eid1805.111366.

Maggi, Ricardo G., Patricia E. Mascarelli, Elizabeth L. Pultorak, Barbara C. Hegarty, Julie M. Bradley, B. Robert Mozayeni, and Edward B. Breitschwerdt. 2011. "*Bartonella* spp. Bacteremia in High-Risk Immunocompetent Patients." *Diagnostic Microbiology and Infectious Disease* 71, no. 4 (December): 430–437. https://doi.org/10.1016/j.diagmicrobio.2011.09.001.

Maluki, Azar, Edward Breitschwerdt, Lynne Bemis, Rosalie Greenberg, Bobak Robert Mozayeni, Jamie Dencklau, and Marna Ericson. 2020. "Imaging Analysis of Bartonella Species in the Skin Using Single-Photon and Multi-Photon (Second Harmonic Generation) Laser Scanning Microscopy." *Clinical Case Reports* 8, no. 8 (August): 1,564–1,570. https://doi.org/10.1002/ccr3.2939.

JIW Marketon and R. Glaser. Stress Hormones and Immune Function. Cellular Immunology Vol 252 Issue 1-2 2008 Pg 16-26.

Mascarelli, Patricia E., Ricardo G. Maggi, Sarah Hopkins, B. Robert Mozayeni, Chelsea L. Trull, Julie M. Bradley, Barbara C. Hegarty, and Edward B. Breitschwerdt. 2013. "*Bartonella henselae* Infection in a Family Experiencing Neurological and Neurocognitive Abnormalities after Woodlouse Hunter Spider Bites." *Parasites & Vectors* 6, no. 98. https://doi.org/10.1186/1756-3305-6-98.

M Drancourt, L Tran-Hung, J Courtin…—The Journal of…, 2005—academic.oup.com. *Bartonella quintana* in a 4000-Year-Old Human Tooth.

Middelveen, Marianne J., Eva Sapi, Jennie Burke, Katherine R. Filush, Agustin Franco, Melissa C. Fesler, and Raphael B. Stricker. 2018. "Persistent *Borrelia* Infection in Patients with Ongoing Symptoms of Lyme Disease." *Healthcare* 6, no. 2 (April 14): 33. https://doi.org/10.3390/healthcare6020033.

Middelveen, Marianne J., Jennie Burke, Eva Sapi, Cheryl Bandoski, Katherine R. Filush, Yean Wang, Agustin Franco, Arun Timmaraju, Hilary A. Schlinger, Peter J. Mayne, and Raphael B. Stricker. 2014. "Culture and Identification of Borrelia Spirochetes in Human Vaginal and Seminal Secretions." *F1000Research*. https://doi.org/10.12688/f1000research.5778.3.

Miklossy, Judith. 2016. "Bacterial Amyloid and DNA are Important Constituents of Senile Plaques: Further Evidence of the Spirochetal and Biofilm Nature of Senile Plaques." *Journal of Alzheimer's Disease* 53, no. 4: 1,459–1,473. https://doi.org/10.3233/JAD-160451.

Miklossy, Judith. 2011. "Alzheimer's Disease—a Neurospirochetosis. Analysis of the Evidence following Koch's and Hill's Criteria." *Journal of Neuroinflammation* 8, article no. 90. https://doi.org/10.1186/1742-2094-8-90.

Miklossy, Judith, Lesley A. Fein, Sherman McCall, Sandor Kasas, and Patrick L. McGeer. 2008. "P1–378: Concurrent Alzheimer's Disease and Lyme Neuroborreliosis: Persisting Atypical Cystic Forms of *Borrelia burgdorferi* in the Brain and Recovery of Cognitive Decline following Antibiotic Treatment." *Alzheimer's & Dementia: The Journal of the Alzheimer's Association*. https://doi.org/10.1016/j.jalz.2008.05.960.

Miklossy, Judith, Sandor Kasas, Anne D. Zurn, Sherman McCall, Sheng Yu, and Patrick L. McGeer. 2008. "Persisting Atypical and Cystic Forms of *Borrelia burgdorferi* and Local Inflammation in Lyme Neuroborreliosis." *Journal of Neuroinflammation* 5, article no. 40. https://doi.org/10.1186/1742-2094-5-40.

Miklossy, Judith, Kamel Khalili, Lise Gern, Rebecca L. Ericson, Pushpa Darekar, Lorie Bolle, Jean Hurlimann, and Bruce J. Paster. 2004. "*Borrelia burgdorferi* Persists in the Brain in Chronic Lyme Neuroborreliosis and May Be Associated with Alzheimer Disease." *Journal of Alzheimer's Disease* 6, no. 6: 639–649. https://doi.org/10.3233/JAD-2004-6608.

Morrissette, Madeleine, Norman Pitt, Antonio González, Philip Strandwitz, Mariaelena Caboni, Alison W. Rebman, Rob

Knight, Anthony D'Onofrio, John N. Aucott, Mark J. Soloski, and Kim Lewis. 2020. "A Distinct Microbiome Signature in Posttreatment Lyme Disease Patients." *mBio* 11, no. 5 (September 29). https://doi.org/10.1128/mBio.02310-20.

Mosel, Michael R., Heather E. Carolan, Alison W. Rebman, Steven Castro, Christian Massire, David J. Ecker, Mark J. Soloski, John N. Aucott, and Mark W. Eshoo. 2019. "Molecular Testing of Serial Blood Specimens from Patients with Early Lyme Disease during Treatment Reveals Changing Coinfection with Mixtures of *Borrelia burgdorferi* Genotypes." *Antimicrobial Agents and Chemotherapy* 63, no. 7 (June 24). https://doi.org/10.1128/AAC.00237-19.

Namrata, Pabbati, Jamie M. Miller, Madari Shilpa, Patlolla R. Reddy, Cheryl Bandoski, Michael J. Rossi, and Eva Sapi. 2014. "Filarial Nematode Infection in *Ixodes scapularis* Ticks Collected from Southern Connecticut." *Veterinary Sciences* 1, no. 1: 5–15. https://doi.org/10.3390/vetsci1010005.

PE Fournier, M Drancourt, G Aboudharam...—Microbes and infection, 2015—Elsevier. Paleomicrobiology of Bartonella infections.

R Barbieri, BHA Mai, T Chenal, ML Bassi, D Gandia...—Scientific reports, 2020—nature.com. [HTML] A 2,000-year-old specimen with intraerythrocytic Bartonella quintana.

Rebman, Alison W., and John N. Aucott. 2020. "Post-Treatment Lyme Disease as a Model for Persistent Symptoms in Lyme Disease." *Frontiers in Medicine* 7 (February 25), article no. 57. https://doi.org/10.3389/fmed.2020.00057.

Rebman, Alison W., Kathleen T. Bechtold, Ting Yang, Erica A. Mihm, Mark J. Soloski, Cheryl B. Novak, and John N. Aucott. 2017. "The Clinical, Symptom, and Quality-of-Life Characterization of a Well-Defined Group of Patients with Posttreatment Lyme Disease Syndrome." *Frontiers in Medicine* 4 (December 14), article no. 224. https://doi.org/10.3389/fmed.2017.00224.

Rudenko, Natalie, Maryna Golovchenko, Katerina Kybicova, and Marie Vancova. 2019. "Metamorphoses of Lyme Disease Spirochetes: Phenomenon of *Borrelia* Persisters." *Parasites &*

Vectors 12, article no. 237 (May 16). https://doi.org/10.1186/
s13071-019-3495-7.

Rudenko, N., M. Golovchenko, M. Vancova, K. Clark, L. Grubhoffer, and J. H. Oliver Jr. 2016. "Isolation of Live *Borrelia burgdorferi* Sensu Lato Spirochaetes from Patients with Undefined Disorders and Symptoms Not Typical for Lyme Borreliosis." *Clinical Microbiology and Infection* 22, no 3: 267. https://doi.org/10.1016/j.cmi.2015.11.009.

Sapi, Eva, Rumanah S. Kasliwala, Hebo Ismail, Jason P. Torres, Michael Oldakowski, Sarah Markland, Gauri Gaur, Anthony Melillo, Klaus Eisendle, Kenneth B. Liegner, Jenny Libien, and James E. Goldman. 2019. "The Long-Term Persistence of *Borrelia burgdorferi* Antigens and DNA in the Tissues of a Patient with Lyme Disease." *Antibiotics* 8, no.4 (October 11): 183. https://doi.org/10.3390/antibiotics8040183.

Sapi, E., K. Balasubramanian, A. Poruri, J. S. Maghsoudlou, K. M. Socarras, A. V. Timmaraju, K. R. Filush, K. Gupta, S. Shaikh, P. A. S. Theophilus, D. F. Luecke, A. MacDonald, B. Zelger. 2016. "Evidence of *In Vivo* Existence of *Borrelia* Biofilm in Borrelial Lymphocytomas." *European Journal of Microbiology and Immunology* 6, no. 1: 9–24. https://doi.org/10.1556/1886.2015.00049.

Sapi, Eva, Scott L. Bastian, Cedric M. Mpoy, Shernea Scott, Amy Rattelle, Namrata Pabbati, Akhila Poruri, Divya Burugu, Priyanka A. S. Theophilus, Truc V. Pham, Akshita Datar, Navroop K. Dhaliwal, Alan MacDonald, Michael J. Rossi, Saion K. Sinha, and David F. Luecke. 2012. "Characterization of Biofilm Formation by *Borrelia burgdorferi In Vitro*." *PLOS ONE* (October 24). https://doi.org/10.1371/journal.pone.0048277.

Sapi, Eva, Navroop Kaur, Samuel Anyanwu, David F. Luecke, Akshita Datar, Seema Patel, Michael Rossi, and Raphael B. Stricker. 2011. "Evaluation of *In Vitro* Antibiotic Susceptibility of Different Morphological Forms of *Borrelia burgdorferi*." *Infection and Drug Resistance* 4 (May 3): 97–113. https://doi.org/10.2147/IDR.S19201.

Borrelia burgdorferi, the causative agent of Lyme disease, forms drug-tolerant persister cells.
B Sharma, AV Brown, NE Matluck, LT Hu… - Antimicrobial agents and Chemotherapy Vol 59 July, 2015 - No. 8

Szczesny, Pawel, Dirk Linke, Astrid Ursinus, Kerstin Bär, Heinz Schwarz, Tanja M. Riess, Volkhard A. J. Kempf, Andrei N. Lupas, Jörg Martin, and Kornelius Zeth. 2008. "Structure of the Head of the *Bartonella* Adhesin BadA." *PLOS Pathogens* (August 8). https://doi.org/10.1371/journal.ppat.1000119.

Theophilus, P. A. S., M. J. Victoria, K. M. Socarras, K. R. Filush, K. Gupta, D. F. Luecke, and E. Sapi. 2015. "Effectiveness of *Stevia rebaudiana* Whole Leaf Extract against the Various Morphological Forms of *Borrelia burgdorferi In Vitro*." *European Journal of Microbiology and Immunology* 5, no. 4: 268–280. https://doi.org/10.1556/1886.2015.00031.

Theophilus, Priyanka A. S., Divya Burugu, Akhila Poururi, Daniel S. Phillips, David F. Luecke. "Effective Antimicrobials for the Different Forms of *Borrelia burgdorferi*."

Timmaraju, Venkata Arun, Priyanka A. S. Theophilus, Kunthavai Balasubramanian, Shafiq Shakih, David F. Luecke, and Eva Sapi. 2015. "Biofilm formation by *Borrelia burgdorferi* Sensu Lato." *FEMS Microbiology Letters* 362, no. 15 (August). https://doi.org/10.1093/femsle/fnv120.

Tsukamoto, Kentaro, Naoaki Shinzawa, Akito Kawai, Masahiro Suzuki, Hiroyasu Kidoya, Nobuyuki Takakura, Hisateru Yamaguchi, Toshiki Kameyama, Hidehito Inagaki, Hiroki Kurahashi, Yasuhiko Horiguchi, and Yohei Doi. 2020. "The *Bartonella* Autotransporter BafA Activates the Host VEGF Pathway to Drive Angiogenesis." *Nature Communications* 11, article no. 3571. https://doi.org/10.1038/s41467-020-17391-2.

Wawrzeniak, Keith, Gauri Gaur, Eva Sapi, and Alireza G. Senejani. 2020. "Effect of *Borrelia burgdorferi* Outer Membrane Vesicles on Host Oxidative Stress Response." *Antibiotics* 9, no. 5: 275. https://doi.org/10.3390/antibiotics9050275.

Weber-Sanders, Melissa, Paulo E. N. F. Velho, Gislaine Vieira-Damiani, Marilene Neves da Silva, Vitor B. Pelegati, Carlos Lenz Cesar, and Marna Ericson. 2015. "*Bartonella henselae* Biofilm Detected on Catheter of Patient with Persistent Bartonellosis." *Microscopy and Microanalysis* 21 (August): 237–238. https://doi.org/10.1017/S1431927615001981.

About the Author

D r. Lesley Ann Fein grew up in South Africa where she attended the University of the Witwatersrand. She completed her bachelor of science degree with an additional year of studies in paleoanthropology and physiology called B.Sc with Honors. She then completed four out of six years of medical school training there.

While in South Africa, she was one of a handful of students who established the Muldersdrift Clinic to provide free medical care to indigent farm laborers. She is very proud that this clinic is now a part of the medical school in Gauteng, previously called Johannesburg.

After coming to the USA, she completed her master's degree in public health at Columbia University, after which she graduated with distinction from George Washington University School of Medicine. She was voted to be a member of AOA and received an award for academic excellence from the American Women's Medical Association. She then completed a residency in Internal Medicine at Mt. Sinai Hospital in NYC and a rheumatology fellowship at NYU.

She has been in private practice in New Jersey since 1988. She became interested in the relationship between infections and autoimmune diseases while at Mt. Sinai, and this passion led to specializing in rheumatology. Throughout her career, she has established a reputation as a diagnostician and was named as one of the top diagnosticians in the U.S. in Medscape.

Since Lyme disease was the first infection documented to trigger a host of autoimmune diseases, she has treated many complicated patients with underlying tick-borne infections manifesting as undiagnosed illnesses, atypical autoimmune disease, fibromyalgia, and

CFS/ME. By the time patients finally see her, they have seen twenty to thirty doctors who have ultimately referred them to a psychiatrist.

Many begin to believe that they are truly crazy. This is the reason for the title of the book. The motivation of this book is to dispel many myths about insect-borne infections and to provide an update on extensive research in the area of Lyme disease and bartonella.

CPSIA information can be obtained
at www.ICGtesting.com
Printed in the USA
JSHW042315150623
43209JS00007B/135

9 781638 605065